Life With a Traumatic Brain Injury:
Finding the Road Back to Normal

Life With a Traumatic Brain Injury:
Finding the Road Back to Normal

by Amy Zellmer

A collection of short stories originally
published on *The Huffington Post*

Published by FuzionPrint
Edited by Connie Anderson
Design by Sue Stein

Cover photo by Amy Zellmer

Life With a Tramatic Brain Injury: Finding the Road Back to Normal
is a work of nonfiction. The names, details,
and circumstances may have been changed to
protect the survivor's identity.

Library of Congress Control Number: 2015917042
ISBN: 9781519101440

Dedicated to My Tribe

Advance Praise for *Life With a Traumatic Brain Injury:*

Amy Zellmer dedicates her book "Life with a TBI: Finding the Road Back to Normal" to her Tribe, and right away I know I'm in good hands. "Speak for us," I hear myself saying out loud. And then more whimsically, "Normal: it's not just a town in Illinois!"

The title and every chapter in Amy's book offer what we need the most, and that is hope. We need hope that there is a road back to normal—our New Normal—and Amy is a reliable, amiable and articulate companion on this strange spooky road with its stops and starts, twists and turns. Through Amy's observations and insights, we see that our destination is not the normal of our old lives back the way they were. With newly compassionate hearts, we also have become cold-eyed realists who see the way more clearly, and we can all thank Amy for taking us along on this hard road. Working together, The Tribe makes sure that better and brighter days are ahead for all of us.

They say that blood is thicker than water, meaning that family ties are, or should be, stronger than mere friendships, but Amy knows something even truer: the bonds within this TBI Tribe are stronger even than family. Too many of us have seen our loved ones' back as they turn away from us. But when you look in the eyes of a survivor, or hear the catch in their throat over the phone, or wait until they have composed themselves after weeping, you know that this person has heard the slammed door, the unspoken goodbyes of abandonment. And you know that this newest member of the Tribe needs you more than they've ever needed anybody.

And so the mutual commitment of Being There is acknowledged and understood.

- John C Byler, Author, *You Look Great! —Strategies for Living Inside a Brain Injury*

Often invisible, TBI takes a toll, not just physically and cognitively, but emotionally and socially, as friendships and empathy are tested "to the max." Amy explains TBI so vividly that the TBI-er feels exonerated, understood, and no longer alone. Those whose loved ones are touched by TBI are given a glimpse and better understanding of their world.

Amy's escape from a dark, lonely place of desperation to a vibrant voice advocating for TBI is an inspiration to all. Her first-person account and collection of personal stories, the factual information, ideas for encouraging and caring for TBI friends and family, and the many resources is incredible on its own merit—but it's truly phenomenal considering it was all written while coping with the challenges of TBI.

—Marlene, Kansas, caregiver-from-afar

My TBI happened thirty-three years ago, there was no information about it back in the eighties. I am so grateful for Amy's book. I recommend that everyone with a TBI, as well as family and friends, read this book. I had no idea that many of my struggles were the result of my TBI—I thought it was just me. Recently I saw a neurologist for the first time, and have finally begun to heal from the emotional turmoil I have been living in because of my TBI. I realized I am not the only one who feels this way. Please read this book and know you are not alone, and seek help for both your mental and physical health. Amy's stories in this book saved me, for I was a breath away from ending my life.

—Becky B., TBI survivor

TABLE OF CONTENTS

Statistics

All information in this section is cited and shared with permission from the Centers for Disease Control and Prevention (cdc.gov).

Overview

Traumatic brain injury (TBI) is a major cause of death and disability in the United States, contributing to about 30 percent of all injury-related deaths. Every day, 138 people in the United States die from injuries that include TBI. Those who survive a TBI can face effects lasting a few days—to disabilities that may last the rest of their lives. Effects of TBI can include impaired thinking or memory, movement, sensation (e.g., vision or hearing), or emotional functioning (e.g., personality changes, depression). These issues not only affect the individual, but can have lasting effects on families and communities.

What is a TBI?

A TBI is caused by a bump, blow, or jolt to the head, or a penetrating head injury that disrupts the normal function of the brain. Not all blows or jolts to the head result in a TBI. The severity of a TBI may range from "mild" (i.e., a brief change in mental status or consciousness) to "severe" (i.e., an extended period of unconsciousness or memory loss after the injury). Most TBIs that occur each year are mild, commonly called concussions. Doctors may describe a concussion as a "mild" brain injury because concussions are usually not life threatening. Even so, their effects   can be serious.

Statistics:

- Every 13 seconds someone in the United States will suffer a TBI.
- Each year a reported 2.5 million people sustain a TBI. 1.365 million people, nearly 80 percent, are treated and released from an emergency department.
- The number of unreported TBIs, or those not seen by a doctor, is unknown.
- Each year, 52,000 people die as a result of a TBI. TBI is a contributing factor to a third (30.5%) of all injury-related deaths in the United States.
- Falls are the leading cause of TBI. Rates are highest for children aged 0 to 4 years, and for adults aged 75 years and older.
- Falls result in the greatest number of TBI-related emergency department visits (523,043) and hospital izations (62,334).
- Motor vehicle-traffic injury is the leading cause of TBI-related death. Rates are highest for adults aged 20 to 24 years.

Foreword

Just a few short years ago, the term Traumatic Brain Injury, was unfamiliar to most. While an estimated 2.5 million Americans sustain a brain injury yearly (Data source: CDC), there was a void in our national narrative about this life-changing epidemic.

Quietly and off the radar screen for most, every day mothers, fathers, sons and daughters, parents and grandparents, are joining an exclusive subset of the population: traumatic brain injury survivors.

In the last few years since I sustained my own brain injury, my story has become part of the national narrative with the publication of my first book, Metamorphosis: Surviving Brain Injury. As time passes, the coverage of brain injury by the mainstream media led one professional at a recent conference I attended to call the media focus on brain injury, "a fevered pitch." And so it should be.

From professional sports lawsuits, to NASCAR drivers, to our troops returning home from overseas, it seems that everywhere you turn, brain injury is finally in the news. The long age of silence that surrounded brain injury is coming to a close.

Over the last few years, I have seen a few rising stars within the brain injury community. Most of these souls are friends, family members, or spouses of someone impacted by traumatic brain injury. Their experiences serve the greater good by keeping TBI in the public spotlight.

But every now and again, an actual brain injury survivor

is left with the unique ability to articulate clearly and concisely what life is like after a brain injury, and does it in a way that those who are affected can understand.

I first heard of Amy Zellmer through her *Huffington Post* pieces. Reading her work through the eyes of a survivor, it was clear that she was writing from the vantage point of being a brain injury survivor herself. Simply put, she was speaking my language. I immediately identified with her experiences as they paralleled my own life. In Amy's new book, she shares many of the triumphs, frustrations, pains, and joys that we within the survivor community face every day.

Amy's work will enlighten and educate those not intimately familiar with the sometimes-subtle nuances of life after a traumatic brain injury.

Better still, as her body of work continues to grow, she will help others, many of whom she will never meet. This I know from personal experiences. And in that selfless helping of others, Amy will continue to lift humanity higher.

—David Grant, author of *Metamorphosis: Surviving Brain Injury* and also *Slices of Life After Traumatic Brain Injury.* David is a staff writer for Brainline.org–a PBS supported web presence, as well as a contributing writer to *Chicken Soup for the Soul: Recovering from Traumatic Brain Injuries.*
David@TBIHopeandInspiration.com
www.TBIHopeandInspiration.com

Acknowledgments

I have so many people to thank, people who influenced and inspired me in profound ways. This book wouldn't be a reality if it weren't for a certain few, and I wish to say a *huge thank you*.

To Jill, my biggest influencer. This book exists only because of your encouragement, and also your seemingly simple statement that I should submit my story to the *Huffington Post*.

To Kjiersten, for knowing from the get-go that this was the path I was meant to be on. Your insight has been a driving force in my writing.

To Laura, for the unconditional love and support, and for knowing all along that everything happens for a reason. You always seem to understand how my mind works, sometimes better than I did.

To Rose, for helping me rehab my broken body with gentle yoga.

To Belinda, for helping me gain back my strength and confidence.

To my parents, who don't always "get" me, but love me unconditionally.

To Marisha and Sherrie, for showing me the way. You may not have realized it, but you have influenced me as a writer in profound ways. I am thrilled to be your neighbor.

To Simon, for always being there for me when I needed comfort—or sushi.

To James and Christie for your experience and guidance throughout this journey.

To Roshini for introducing me to Connie Anderson and the Women of Words (WOW) writing group. Without you two, I most definitely know this book wouldn't be a reality (at least not yet). And to Connie for her editing and book-related guidance.

To my fellow ambassadors with the Brain Injury Association of America, and with the Minnesota TBI Advisory Committee, as well as the staff and volunteers at the Minnesota Brain Injury Alliance. *Awareness is growing.*

To Toni P., Paul B., Stephanie F., Anne F., April I., Heather S., Jennifer W., Amy P., John B., Lynn J., and all of my fellow survivors who at great lengths have supported me as an advocate. You know how to lift me up when I am down, and remind me of my passion and mission. #SurvivorsRock

To Peter, Sarah, Rick, and all of my Kickstarter backers, for your generous pledges to my Kickstarter campaign. Your support has allowed this book to go forth into the world in order to create awareness.

To Drs. Fred, Bob, and Greg, for your keen attention to my injuries, as well as your unconditional support. There is nothing more important for a doctor to say than, "You're going to get through this!"

INTRODUCTION

What began as a blog post on my personal blog led to something bigger than I could have ever imagined. When my friend suggested I submit it to *Huffington Post*, I almost didn't. I did not think that my story would be of any interest to anyone other than me. Boy, was I wrong. I am eternally thankful to Jill for giving me that extra nudge to submit it.

As I sat at my computer and watched my first published piece go live, I was hoping that at least a few people would read it. If I were able to help just one other person dealing with TBI, then my efforts would be worth it. What I witnessed still amazes me. It started with 500 likes, then 1,000, then 10,000. My story had officially gone viral. As of today, over 30,000 people have liked, shared, tweeted, pinned, and commented on my original post. My book is named after this original, viral piece.

Other survivors have sent hundreds of emails, tweets, and Facebook messages, thanking me for putting into words how they felt. They were sharing my story with their family and friends so that these people could better understand what their loved one was going through. It was at this point that I knew I had stumbled onto something. There was a huge void in the TBI world, and I could use my words to help fill it.

The private Facebook group I created, which I affectionately named The TBI Tribe, became a place where we could all hang out and share what we were going through. It is currently up to almost 3,000 members, comprised of survivors and their loved ones. The Tribe is what keeps me motivated to write as they encourage and support me every step of the way. They are the people I turn to when I need some extra inspiration or a few quotes for my story.

This book is comprised of short stories, most of which were originally published on *Huffington Post*. They have also been shared on other sites such as BrainLine.org, Vivid & Brave, The Good Men Project, and TBI Hope and Inspiration.

I want this book to help raise awareness about this invisible injury that affects so many—and to bring hope to survivors, and understanding to their loved ones.

Part One:
Life With a Traumatic Brain Injury

Split Seconds

by Amy Zellmer

I am lost in the darkness,
Not sure which way to turn.
I think I can see a light…
But it's out of my grasp.

Thoughts spiraling in my head
Unsure of where I belong.
Nothing makes sense anymore…
I'm sure I was wrong.

Everything is twisting,
Turning and spinning.
What I once thought was normal—
Has been turned upside down.

We never think it can happen to us
The unthinkable words that we hear.
It's a simple accident—
and our world is changed in split seconds.

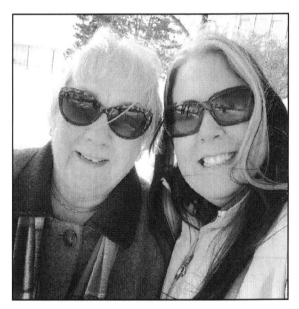

My mom with me the day before I fell

Chapter 1

The Day My Life Changed

February 2015

A Little Backstory

As I neared the one-year mark since my accident, I had been thinking about writing a blog post on it. Actually, I had thought a lot about it the entire past year. But I didn't. I didn't have the courage. I've been scared. Scared of what people might think. Scared that people will be snarky or rude. Scared of what I might feel. Scared of reliving the fall. Scared that no one will read it. Then I heard a voice in my head say, "Screw it! Writing is your therapy, Amy. It's time to write it down, and get it out of your head!"

If my story can inspire even just one person, it is so worth getting past my fear, so here goes.

My Story

It's been almost a year since that cold February day in 2014 that I slipped on a patch of sheer ice in my building's driveway, and landed smack on my head. I can still feel my feet slipping out from under me, knowing there was *absolutely nothing* I could do as both feet went straight up in the air (I imagine I looked a bit like a cartoon). I can still hear the terrible, god-awful sound of my skull making impact with the concrete. I can still remember thinking to myself, "Oh, no. This is *not good.*" I can still remember sitting up and finding Pixxie, my eight-pound Yorkie, tail tucked under, looking at me like "What the heck just happened, Mom?" I remember the excruciating pain on the back my head, and the swirling, flickering lights in my peripheral vision.

We (my team of doctors and me) are pretty certain that I blacked out for at least a few minutes. I had been holding Pixxie in my left arm when I fell. Given she was about seven feet away when I sat up, she had had some time during which she got up and walked away from me. Who knows, maybe she even sat there and licked my face for five minutes. No one was around, and security cameras don't capture that part of our parking lot. I will never know for sure: Did I lay there limp and helpless for seconds—or minutes?

We think that my body reacted instinctively and protected Pixxie like a baby, and that is why my arms didn't go down to break the fall, causing my skull to take the full impact. Let me say that again: *My skull took the full impact of the fall.* The resulting injuries, as diagnosed by my chiropractor and neurologist, included: a severe concussion, mild traumatic brain injury (TBI), torn/pulled muscles in my neck, throat, abdomen, and chest, and a dislocated sternum. I hurt in places I didn't even know it was possible to hurt.

In the days to follow, I think if I heard one more person say. "*It's just a concussion,*" I may have punched them. Concussions often lead to TBIs, and are quite serious. Every concussion is a brain injury, to some extent.

According to the Centers for Disease Control and Prevention (CDC):

- Approximately 2.5 million people in the U.S. suffer from a traumatic brain injury each year.
- 52,000 people die from TBI each year.
- 85,000 people suffer long-term disabilities.
- In the U.S., more than 5.3 million people live with disabilities caused by TBI.

Yes, *people die* from falls like the one I took, but somehow I came away with my life. For that, I am forever grateful.

Now, one year later, I…

- Am still struggling with the effects of my TBI, as well as all of my physical injuries.
- Have felt an entire spectrum of emotions: anger, rage, fear, sadness, depression, hope, joy, frustration, and contentment.
- Struggle with being in crowded restaurants or shopping malls.
- Can't handle over-stimulation from multiple sources (light, sound, vibration).
- Get confused easily.
- Forget things in seconds, but can remember them days later.
- Suffer from constant vertigo and dizziness.
- Am up and down emotionally, like a speeding roller

coaster.
- Am exhausted beyond comprehension.
- Grab for words that seem to have disappeared into thin air.
- Have noticed that my personality has changed, and I am aware of my mood swings.
- Have anxiety and panic attacks—which scared the crap out of me when they first happened.
- Have some really good days—and I have some really bad days.

When I wake up in the morning, I say a little prayer that it's going to be a good day, because sometimes *the bad days are just more than I can handle.*

People make assumptions that I must be fine because mine is an "invisible injury," and they see me constantly working my butt off trying to continue making a living. What they don't see is:
- My pain and exhaustion at the end of the day.
- The consecutive days spent in bed because I physically don't have the strength and energy to do anything.
- The ice packs, ibuprofen, and the hot baths with Epsom salts.
- The rescheduled sessions and missed hours of work.
- The massages, physical therapy, and the PTSD therapy sessions.
- The seventy-some doctor visits in ten months.

They also don't see the uncertainty of whether I'll be able

to continue as a photographer, which is a much more physically and mentally challenging career than most people realize. But I have no choice other than to power through it, and keep on working. As a single woman who is self-employed and living on her own, the financial struggle has been very real, and frightening at times. What little I had saved was eaten up after my divorce a few years ago. I am not complaining. It's all been working out just fine. But I truly want people to fully understand my struggle—physically, emotionally, mentally, and financially.

When I wasn't able to get out of the bathtub one night shortly after I fell, I realized that I needed some help and support. I decided to go stay with my parents for a few weeks. During that time, it was comforting to be around them, and know that they were there in case I needed anything. Being alone in my loft gave me an overpowering sense of loneliness that I most certainly needed to escape. I am quite independent, and tend to overdo things, so this has been a great lesson in patience, and in asking for help.

Now, I am not telling you all of this to make you feel pity for me. Far from it. I want you to understand that this invisible illness is very real. Because there are so many of us in your community, chances are you will run into someone with a TBI on your next trip to the store, at your job, or walking/driving on the road along side you. Next time the person in front of you at the grocery store is having a hard time counting out her money, or is walking a little too slowly in front of you, or can't remember what he was saying to you mid-sentence, or is staring blankly at the shelves with her cart in the middle of the aisle, please, have some grace. We can't help it. It is who we are now. Every day the journey gets easier, but there's a very real chance that it will never go away completely. Every single day someone commits suicide because he or she can't cope with the chronic struggles of a TBI. I do not want to be one of those people.

Please! Don't ever say to a person who has just had a head injury, "It's just a concussion. You'll be fine." That is not what we want to hear, and it's simply not the truth. Instead, offer to bring us a meal or run some errands. I couldn't figure out how to use my microwave, let alone my oven, after my accident, and I had no idea how to use the ATM at the bank.

Offer them your ear and/or shoulder (I thought Bill Clinton was still our president). Show them that you care—because we are in a very dark and lonely place. While you can never understand what it's like to live with a TBI, you can show compassion and empathy. Instead of asking, "How are you feeling?" ask, "What can I do for you?" Also, don't make fun of the situation. I remember on several occasions when people said things like, "Well, you shouldn't be wearing stilettos out in the ice," or "Sounds like you need to wear a helmet in your parking lot," or "Were you attempting Crashed Ice?" These attempts at humor were not at all funny in the days after a traumatic accident. Not to mention that brain injuries can cause you to be very emotional at every little thing. (I still cry when I see a stupid cat video on YouTube). *Also, I want to clarify that I was wearing winter boots when I fell, not stilettos.*

I am eternally grateful for a friend who offered to spend that first night at my house after I fell. I was terrified of going to sleep that night, and it was comforting to know that he was downstairs if I needed him. I am grateful for the friend who brought me fruit, and made me chili. I am grateful for the friends who called to show they cared, and asked if I needed anything. I am grateful for the doctor with a positive attitude who continually reassured me that I would get through this. I am grateful for assistants who jumped in to help me when I needed it. I am independent and stubborn, so it was very hard for me to sit back and accept all of this support. But without it, I truly may not be here today.

Situations like these can cause some friendships to end, but also new friendships to form. I am thankful for the amazing people who have come into my life since my accident. The universe has given me more than I thought I was capable of handling, only to prove to me that I am a lot stronger than I ever thought. I have learned to slow down, honor my body, give myself grace, and know that everything will be okay. I know that everything happens for a reason, and there is a reason the universe wanted me to experience this. I am grateful for the lessons I am learning from this, and the ones that I have yet to figure out. One day at a time, one foot in front of the other. When the going gets tough, really tough, you gotta keep on going.

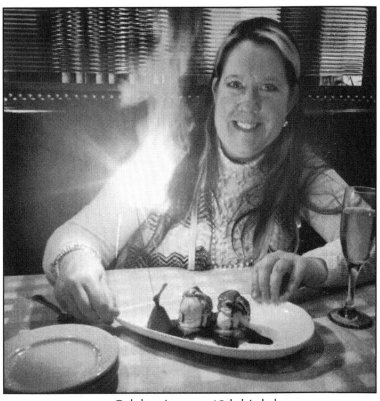

Celebrating my 40th birthday
one month after my fall

Chapter 2

Life With a TBI: March is National Brain Injury Awareness Month

March 2015

Last year at this time, I was enduring the beginning of my life with a TBI, while approaching my fortieth birthday. I had no idea that March was National Brain Injury Awareness Month. This year I feel compelled to shout it from the rooftops, or the computer screen, with stories about the journeys of those living with a traumatic brain injury (TBI), or who are caring for a loved one who is recovering from one. My hope is to educate those who aren't familiar with TBI, and to help other TBI-ers understand that they are not alone, and that their symptoms are not just "in their head" (pun intended).

Let me start by offering you some statistics on TBI from BrainTrauma.org:

- Traumatic brain injury (TBI) is the leading cause of death and disability in children and adults from ages 1 to 44.
- Brain injuries are most often caused by motor vehicle crashes, sports injuries—or simple falls on the play-
- ground, at work, or in the home.

- Every year, approximately 52,000 deaths occur from traumatic brain injury.
- An estimated 1.6 million to 3.8 million sports-related TBIs occur each year.
- At least 5.3 million Americans, 2 percent of the U.S. population, currently live with disabilities resulting from TBI.
- Moderate and severe head injury (respectively) is associated with a 2.3 and 4.5 times increased risk of Alzheimer's disease.
- Males are about twice as likely as females to experience a TBI.
- Exposures to blasts are a leading cause of TBI among active duty military personnel in war zones.
- Veterans' advocates believe that between 10 and 20 percent of Iraq veterans have some level of TBI.
- About 30 percent of soldiers admitted to Walter Reed Army Medical Center have been diagnosed as having had a TBI.
- The number of people with TBI who are not seen in an emergency department, or who receive no care, is unknown.

There are three levels of traumatic brain injuries: mild, moderate, and severe. Don't let these names fool you. A mild TBI is as serious as a moderate or severe one. The names refer to loss of consciousness and mental alteration as a result of the trauma. In my case, we think I was unconscious for only about a minute or so, therefore classifying me as "mild." However, the resulting damage can be the same for all three because a *TBI does not discriminate.*

A TBI changes you—literally and figuratively. My personality is different. My energy levels and sleep patterns are foreign to me. The confused woman in the kitchen staring at the oven is someone I am now finally starting to understand. The woman who has to write a sticky note for every single task on her to-do list is no longer the multi-tasker she once was. The woman who used to type at 100 words per minute, with zero mistakes, now has to take her time and correct many errors as she types because her brain gets confused with letters.

I am finally coming to terms with this "new me." It has been over a year since I fell on the ice, landing full force on my skull. In the beginning I was angry. I was confused. I was in a lot of pain, both physically and emotionally. People didn't understand, and they didn't believe me because they couldn't understand my hidden injuries. I didn't have a strong support system—but what I did have was determination.

Life with an "invisible" injury or illness can be a real challenge. Since I posted my blog, "Life With a Traumatic Brain Injury," on *The Huffington Post,* I have made an entirely new circle of friends. I created a group on Facebook, affectionately named "The TBI Tribe." This is a safe place where we can hang out, talk, vent our frustrations, share in each other's successes, and more importantly, have a place where we all feel like we fit in. I was craving an environment where others understood my struggles, and who didn't pass judgment. I have found exactly that in this tribe of others on the same journey.

I want to share with you a little bit about one of my new friends, Jennifer L. White from St. Louis, Missouri.

In July of 2000 Jennifer collapsed in her Atlanta, Georgia apartment. She called 911 and told them she was dying. She did, in fact, die in the ambulance on her way to the hospital. Fortunately medics were able to resuscitate her. Doctors determined that she had had a stroke, and performed brain surgery to eradicate the brain bleed. She spent ten days in the ICU, followed by several months in a rehab facility. Overnight she went from the vice president of a large marketing firm, to being unemployable and on disability. The massive stroke has left Jennifer with cognitive deficiencies, balance issues, and double vision. She jokes that she can, however, make a killer peanut butter sandwich. It's important to have a good sense of humor when dealing with a TBI. Aside from her impairments, Jennifer looks completely healthy and "normal." Jennifer added:

"The brain injury has affected me in a variety of ways. Emotionally, I am fragile, but working hard to toughen my spirit. I am much more introspective (I don't know if this is from the actual brain injury or the fact I now have more time to be introspective). Things are much harder for me than most people. I have to actually seriously think about where I am stepping. I define my life in two ways: before and after the stroke. It has certainly delivered me a tough blow. I have been advised not to have children. I am scared that I am predisposed to have something else happen to me. I don't find sweetness in the sweet things in life because I am more bitter than I want to be—and this makes me sad. But call me crazy... I am glad to be alive."

Life with a TBI truly is a roller coaster ride. I know that my fall could have killed me, and I am thankful every day to be alive, and help bring awareness to the world about TBI.

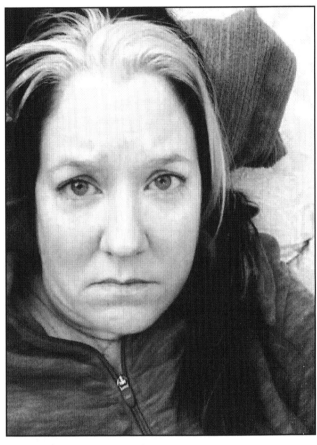

This is me, several days after my fall,
feeling like I had been run over by a truck.

Chapter 3

Five Things Every TBI Survivor
Wants You to Understand

March 2015

To help educate others and bring awareness, please understand that:

1. Our brains no longer work the same.

We have cognitive deficiencies that don't make sense, even to us. Some of us struggle to find the right word, while others can't remember what they ate for breakfast. People who don't understand, including some who are close to us, get annoyed with us and think we're being "flaky" or not paying attention. This couldn't be further from the truth because we have to try even harder to pay attention to things because we know we have deficiencies.

Susan from Lansing, Michigan, suffered a TBI in May of 2013 after the car she was a passenger in hit a tree at 50 mph. She sums up her "new brain" with these words:

"Almost two years post-accident, I still suffer short-term memory loss and language/speech problems. I have learned to write everything down immediately, or else it is more than likely the information is gone and cannot be retrieved. My brain sometimes does not allow my mouth to speak the words that I am trying to get out."

2. We suffer a great deal of fatigue.

We may seem "lazy" to those who don't understand, but the reality is that our brains need *a lot more sleep* than normal, healthy brains. We also have crazy sleep patterns, sometimes sleeping only three hours each night—those hours between 1 and 5 a.m. are very lonely when you're wide awake—and at other times, sleeping up to 14 hours each night. These nights are usually after exerting a lot of physical or mental energy.

Every single thing we do, whether physical or mental, takes a toll on our brain. The more we use it, the more it needs to rest. If we go out to a crowded restaurant with a lot of noise and stimulation, we may simply get over-loaded, and need to go home and rest. Even reading or watching TV causes our brains to fatigue.

Toni P. from Alexandria, Virginia, has sustained multiple TBIs from three auto accidents, her most recent one being in 2014. She sums up fatigue perfectly:

"I love doing things others do, however my body does not appreciate the strain and causes me to "pay the price," which is something that others don't see. I like to describe that my cognitive/physical energy is like a change jar. Everything I do costs a little something out of the jar. If I keep taking money out of the jar, without depositing anything back into the jar, eventually I run out of energy. I just don't know when this will happen. Sometimes it's from an activity that seemed very simple, but was more work then I intended. For me, like others with TBIs, I'm not always aware of it until after I've done too much."

3. We live with fear and anxiety.

Many of us live in the constant state of fear of hurting ourselves again. Yes, I have a fear of falling on the ice, and in general, of hitting my head. I know I suffered a very hard blow to my head, and I am not sure exactly how much it can endure if I were to injure it again. I am deeply afraid that if it were to take another blow, I may not recover, or I may find myself completely disabled, or possibly die. I am fortunate to have a great understanding of the Law of Attraction, and with the help of a therapist, I am trying my hardest to change my fears into positive thoughts.

Other survivors have a daily struggle of even trying to get out of bed in the morning. They are terrified of what might happen next to them. Many TBI survivors live with these legitimate fears. For many, it manifests into anxiety. Some have such profound anxiety that they can hardly leave their home.

Jason Donarski-Wichlacz from Duluth, Minnesota, received a TBI in December of 2014 after being kicked in the head by a patient in a behavioral health facility. He speaks of his struggles with anxiety:

"I never had anxiety before, but now I have panic attacks every day. Sometimes they are about my future and will I get better, will my wife leave me, am I still a good father. Other times it is because matching my socks is overwhelming, or someone ate the last peanut butter cup. I am easily startled and jump at almost everything. I can send my wife a text when she is in the same room, so I know her phone is going to chime... Still I jump every time it chimes. Grocery stores are terrifying. All the colors, the stimulation, and words everywhere. I get overwhelmed, and can't remember where anything is, or what I came for."

4. We deal with chronic pain.

Many of us sustained multiple injuries in our accidents. Once the broken bones are healed, and the bruises and scars have faded, we still deal with a lot of chronic pain. I suffered a considerable amount of neck and chest damage. This pain is sometimes so bad that I am not able to get comfortable enough in bed in order to fall asleep. Others have constant migraines from having hit their head. For most of us, a change in weather wreaks all sort of havoc on our bodies.

Monica, of Los Angeles, California, fell on to concrete

while having a seizure in 2011, fracturing her skull, and resulting in a TBI. She speaks about her chronic migraine headaches
(which are all too common for TBI survivors):

"I never had migraines until I sustained a head injury.
Now I have one, or sometimes a cluster of two or three,
every few weeks. They also crop up when I am stressed
or sleep deprived. Sometimes medication works like
magic, but other times I have to wait out the pain. When
the migraine is over, I am usually exhausted and spacey
for a day or two."

5. We often feel isolated and alone.

Because of all the issues stated above, we sometimes have
a hard time leaving the house. Recently I attended a get-
together of friends at a restaurant. There were TVs all
over the room, all on different channels. The lights were
dim, and there was a lot of buzz from all of the talking. I
had a very hard time concentrating on what anyone at
our table was saying, and the constantly changing lights
on the TVs were simply too much for me to bear. It was
sensory stimulation overload. I lasted about two hours
before I had to go home and collapse into bed.

My friends don't see that part. They don't understand
what it's like. This is what causes many of us to feel so
isolated and alone. The "invisible" aspect of what we deal
with on a daily basis is a lonely struggle.

Kirsten from San Francisco, California, fell while ice-skat-
ing about a year ago, and sustained a TBI. She speaks so per-

fectly to the feelings of depression and isolation:

> "Even though my TBI was a "mild" one, I found myself dealing with a depression that was two-fold. I was not only depressed because of my new mental and physical limitations, but also because many of my symptoms forced me to spend long periods of time self-isolating from the things—like social interactions—that would trigger problems for me. With TBI, it is very easy to get mentally and emotionally turned inward, which is a very lonely place to be."

TBI manifests itself differently within each individual survivor, yet we all seem to experience similarities. At its core, all we ask is that everyone treat each other with human compassion, and don't be so quick to judge one another. You never know what invisible struggle they are dealing with.

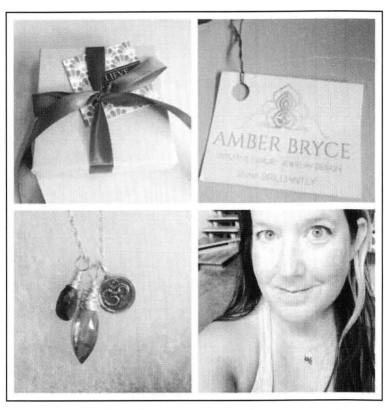

My dear friend, Amber Bryce, created an amazing healing energy necklace for me to wear during my recovery

Chapter 4

Life With a TBI: What I Wish I Had Known When I First Hit My Head

March 2015

There are so many things I wish I had known when I first fell on that patch of ice, landing directly on my skull. I will never be able to clear the sound of the "thud" from my head. I knew from the excruciating pain I was experiencing at the impact point on my head that it was bad, *real bad*. It is my scar, my reminder of how quickly life can change, but I had no idea *how it would change.*

I consider myself fortunate to have found a doctor right away who specializes in head injuries and concussions. However, I feel there are still many things that could have done differently to prepare me for the unexpected roller coaster ride I was now getting on. I hadn't yet even buckled the proverbial seatbelt, in terms of what I was about to experience.

I remember the first day pretty vividly. I fell at about 8 a.m., and was at the doctor's office by 10 a.m. He checked me over and told me I had a severe concussion, and had also torn a few muscles in my neck, throat, and chest. Oddly, I didn't feel any pain other than what felt like a knife stabbing into my skull. It hadn't even occurred to me yet that I had other physical injuries. Actually it was almost two full days before the pain set in, and then it felt like I had been run over by a truck.

I noticed many cognitive deficiencies right away the first day I fell. I was told that this was "normal," and I should start to see improvement in six to eight weeks. So as I neared the end of the eighth week, I was starting to panic. "What's wrong with me? Why am I not getting better? Is there something seriously wrong?" I was experiencing a great deal of confusion, and I was having a lot of trouble finding the word I was looking for, and you could hear in my speech that I was taking longer to complete sentences than I should. My doctor finally sent me to a neurologist who ordered an MRI to rule out anything more severe. It wasn't until this point that anyone started talking about TBI. Even then, I was told it could take a few months to improve; however, at the six-month mark, I was told it could even take up to a year or longer.

What I wish more than anything was that my doctors had been more forthcoming. I understand that every brain injury is different, and not everyone will suffer the same symptoms and time frames. However, in hindsight, it is pretty clear to me that six to eight weeks isn't a realistic timeline. I don't doubt my doctor's abilities, and I know he was trying to do me a "favor" by telling me I'd be fine in no time. But the truth is— I think he was damaging my recovery efforts by doing so.

I also wish I had been sent to occupational therapy right away. The neurologist brought it up, stating that perhaps we should wait, but nothing ever came of it. I wasn't in a proper state of mind to advocate for my health in the way that I normally would. I didn't have a caregiver or spouse living with me who could advocate either. I was alone in my journey. As I look back at those first eight months or so, I see how foggy and dazed I truly was. I encourage you to take an advocate with you to your appointments, even if you don't think it is necessary.

When I reached the six-month mark of my recovery, I started experiencing more dizziness and balance issues than I had been having previously. I started having anxiety because I didn't know what was wrong with me. I was worried that I should be getting better because that is what the doctor had said. I was thrown into a very dark, lonely place. I was starting to become depressed, which was a new experience. I knew I was depressed, yet I didn't know what to do about it. I had no one in my support system to turn to. I felt very isolated and alone.

This cycle of despair went on for about three or four more months, and then I had a complete and total panic attack. I honestly thought I was having a heart attack. My heart was racing, my body felt like it was floating, I wanted to cry and scream, but I had no idea why. Fortunately a dear friend was home when I called, and she helped me calm down. She knew what was happening, as she had experienced panic attacks herself. I was left feeling shaken and scared. "What is wrong with me?" I kept wondering.

The next day I spoke to my doctor about what had happened. He assured me that this was "normal," and part of the recovery process. He was expecting it, as he knew that it would eventually happen to me, and was surprised it had taken me this long to have one. This was yet another thing I wish I had known about, as it would have saved me from the deep sense of fear I had been feeling during the panic attack. Fortunately since that night, I have not had another full-blown attack. I have occasions where I feel the anxiety creeping up, but I am now able to fight it off using deep breathing and meditation.

Finally, thirteen months after my fall, and I am *now* starting physical therapy for my injuries, and occupational therapy for my cognitive issues. I feel like I am late to the party where I should have been months ago. Late is better than never, but I'm not one to be fashionably late.

I wish I had known so many other things in the beginning, and the list could go on and on. I realize that our doctors can't predict the future, or know exactly what is happening inside our brains. Again, I feel blessed to have found a doctor right away who understood concussions and TBI. My wish is that more doctors would begin to understand the true complexity of TBI, no matter how seemingly innocent the concussion appears at first. Patients and caregivers value and appreciate knowing.

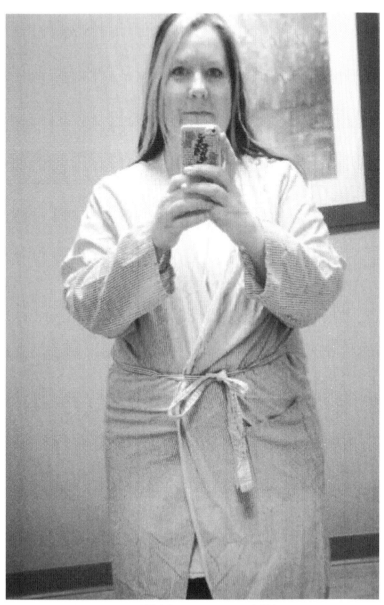

Waiting to get my MRI

Chapter 5

Life With a TBI: Please
Don't Think I'm a Flake

March 2015

I was walking down the inclined driveway at my apartment building when I slipped on a patch of sheer ice, and landed smack on the back of my skull, and was knocked out for a short period of time. When I started to come around, I saw the proverbial stars in my vision, and was totally and completely dazed and confused. If it weren't for a good friend who advised me to go to a specific doctor who specializes in concussions, I am not quite sure what I might have done. Anyone who has just taken a severe blow to the head is in no position to make any major decisions—not to mention I probably shouldn't have driven.

I left my doctor's office and attempted to use the ATM at my bank, I had absolutely no idea what I was supposed to do with my card. Later that evening I attempted to use my microwave and there were far too many buttons, I couldn't understand how to make it work. It was scary....

These simple things I used to do every day without thinking, now required relearning and major effort.

Here I am a year later, I still have a lot of cognitive issues, such as finding the right word, mixing up words, and short-term memory problems. The more fatigued or stressed I am, the worse the symptoms become. In addition to these cognitive problems, I have a lot of issues with over-stimulation as well as being in low-light environments. I also get confused easily when in an unfamiliar place, or when I am forced to make quick decisions.

It is frustrating, to say the least, when my friends get annoyed because I forgot mid sentence what I was telling them, or completely forget a gathering we were supposed to have. If I don't answer a text message or email right away, there is a strong chance that I will completely forget about it, and thus I never answer it. I have repeatedly told my friends what my symptoms and problem areas are, yet they think I am being a flake. They simply don't understand. Or perhaps they are afraid to face the situation at hand—*the uncomfortable fact that I have suffered a brain injury.*

There are times when I pull up Google on my computer to look up something specific. By the time the page is loaded, I have forgotten what it was that I needed to look up. It is incredibly frustrating for me, and for friends to indicate that I might be faking this doesn't help the situation any.

When I lose the word I was going to say, or get up to do something and forget halfway there what I was doing, please don't say to me, "Oh, I do that all the time, too!" I can't differentiate if you're saying this in an attempt to mean well, or if you're trying to say that there's actually nothing wrong with me—because there is. Before my fall, like everyone, I sometimes forgot what I was going to do. However, my experiences now are totally and completely different. My mind is blank, a literal black hole. I can't recall the information. It's gone. POOF!

Amy Pilotte from Manchester, New Hampshire, sustained a TBI in July of 2014 after being rear-ended at a stop sign. She explains how the cognitive issues have changed her:

> "I cannot stay focused. I can't complete a task if it involves more than a few steps. I'm easily overwhelmed and distracted. My memory works when it feels like working, and not a moment sooner."

When I tell you at the last minute that I am not feeling 100 percent, and won't be able to make it to your event, please don't get upset with me. When I wake up in the morning, I don't always know right away what kind of day it's going to be. Many days start out fine, but go downhill quickly. The brain fog rolls in, the headache emerges, and complete fatigue takes over, or my physical pains get the best of me. Some days I am easily over-stimulated. If you have invited me out to a crowded restaurant where I know there will be a lot of noise and dim lighting, I may choose to stay home instead of fighting to understand a word you're saying to me.

It is hurtful when people in my life tell me I'm being flakey or flighty, or that what I am experiencing is a part of "getting older." I wish they would take a moment to truly understand what I am going through, what it is like to live with my traumatic brain injury...every single day. I don't like being this way, but it is who I am now, and I have come to accept it.

It is my mission to help bring awareness to the world about TBI, and be a voice for the many survivors who cannot or do not speak out about their experiences.

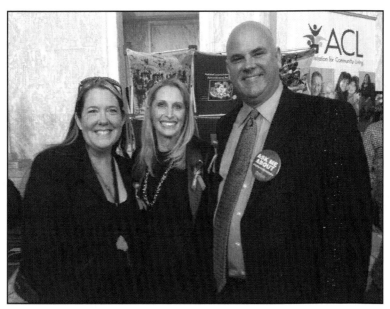

In Washington, D.C. with Stephanie
Freeman and Paul Bosworth

Chapter 6

Brain Injury Awareness Day
in Washington, D.C.

April 2015

In March 2015, I had attended Brain Injury Awareness Day at our national's capitol in Washington, D.C. My journey began in mid-February when my story, "Life With a Traumatic Brain Injury," was published on *The Huffington Post*. I had finally mustered up the courage to share my story with the world, and had two hopes: 1) Maybe, just maybe, one person would read it and be inspired by it, knowing he or she is not alone in this journey. 2) Or maybe it would help educate one, ten or a hundred persons on what living with a traumatic brain injury is like.

After the story went live, I received hundreds of emails and Facebook messages from other survivors sharing their stories with me, thanking me *for putting into words* what they hadn't been able to articulate. Each one was sharing my story with family and friends in an effort to help them understand what these survivors feel emotionally and physically while dealing with a TBI.

This led me to create a Facebook group for survivors and caregivers, which I affectionately named "The TBI Tribe." In my next *Huffington Post* piece, I mentioned this new group. Within a few days I had over 300 members in my group, and one person invited me to come out to Washington, D.C. for Brain Injury Awareness Day on Capitol Hill. I was thrilled and honored, but it was less than two weeks away, and I simply didn't have the funds to go. After some encouragement from several members of the group and a close friend, I decided to try a GoFundMe crowd-sourcing campaign to see if I could raise enough money to cover my travel expenses.

What happened next is truly amazing. I am in awe of the generosity and support of so many. Complete strangers were donating to my cause because they had faith and trust in me to be their voice for TBI awareness. Along with complete strangers, numerous friends also contributed to my campaign, and in less than a week I had enough money to purchase my plane ticket and pay for my hotel room, as well as cover ground transportation costs and food. I was truly blown away. This tribe of mine truly inspires me in ways that they will never understand.

What the tribe doesn't realize is how much they have helped me heal, and also to understand that I am not alone in this journey. Knowing that the symptoms and struggles I have been having are "normal" has really helped me move forward. Up until this point, I had been scared and confused about my future, now I am confident that great things are quickly approaching, and that my healing will only continue to get better. Their words of encouragement and love keep me writing and advocating for awareness.

My day on Capitol Hill was magical and eye opening. I was

unaware of so many of the resources available to help us TBI survivors. Paul Bosworth, a member of my tribe, was particularly helpful in preparing me for my trip to D.C. He prepped me on what information to bring, and what to say when I met with my legislators.

The day started with breakfast with my Minnesota Senator, Al Franken. I also had some time to chat with his aide, Erika, and left her a packet of information on brain injury, as well as printouts of my *Huffington Post* blogs.

Additionally, I met an amazing group of women from Minnesota who were there for colorectal awareness, one of whom has a husband who is a neurologist in the Minneapolis-St. Paul area. I believe everything happens for a reason, and our paths were meant to cross. I can't wait to connect with these women when we are all back in Minnesota.

After breakfast, I spent several hours in the trade show. I met with about fifty different vendors, spending a lot of time talking with them and telling them my story. It was touching how sincerely they wanted to hear our stories, and many of them also had their own TBI story. I had the pleasure to meet a handful of people from my tribe, including Toni, who originally invited me and started this whole journey. Additionally, I met Noel and Kelly from Brain Line, who have generously shared all of my *Huffington Post* blogs on their site, including "5 Things Every TBI Survivor Wants You to Understand," which has gone viral. It was such a pleasure to get to meet the faces behind the page.

It was then time to head to the official briefing with Congressman Bill Pascrell, Jr. (D) of New Jersey. My favorite quote of his was "every concussion is brain injury!" This is a powerful statement, as so many people think a concussion is "no big deal," when in fact every time you get a concussion, you are getting some level of brain trauma and injury.

We also heard from Mac Fedge, a thirteen-year survivor, and his mom, Kathy. They focused on the fact that our health care system needs to change, and also to grasp a better understanding of TBI. Kathy was told that Mac would "be a vegetable" for the rest of his life, and insurance cut him off after a year or two, stating that he was never going to get better. Let's just say that Mac and his family totally proved them wrong. Injured when he was nineteen, now in his early thirties, while Mac still has his struggles, he can now talk, read, play chess, and give a presentation.

We also heard from Matt Breiding, Ph.D., Commander, U.S. Public Health Service Commissioned Corps, and David Williamson, M.D., Neuropsychiatrist & Medical Director, Inpatient Traumatic Brain Injury Program, Walter Reed National Military Medical Center.

A few of the biggest take-aways for me were:
- The CDC has finally updated their statistics on TBI after almost 10 years;
- Healing of the brain can continue to happen for years, and it's a slow process for some people; and
- Aspects of us will never return to the way we were.

For us TBI'ers, it is all about "Finding the New Normal!"

After the amazing lineup of speakers, there was a lovely reception for us, after which I had to head to the airport to return home. It was a fantastic experience, and I am forever grateful that my friends and Tribe afforded me this opportunity. I returned home exhausted, but energized and inspired. I can't wait for next year.

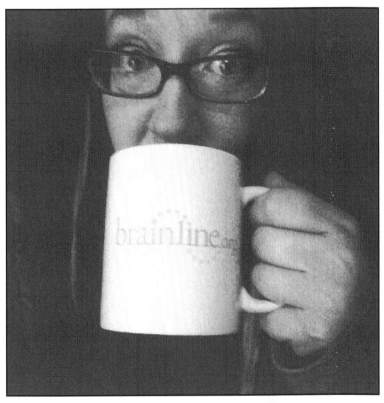

Enjoying my morning coffee
out of my brainline.org mug

Chapter 7

Lost: Life With a TBI

June 2015

Yesterday I got lost driving home from the Target that I visit frequently. I was driving the same route that I always take, yet, all of a sudden, nothing looked familiar, and panic set in. Where the heck was I? How did I get here?

Getting lost and/or confused is my "new normal." Fortunately, I no longer burst into tears and crawl into bed for three days after an instance such as this. I have learned to understand my limits, and know that this kind of thing is going to disrupt my daily life from here on out. It's the way that it is, for now.

The good news is that I have a smartphone. When I do get lost, I pull up my map and find my way home. Usually once I get back on track, I realize where I am, and can navigate my way without further incident.

What's especially frustrating is that if you knew me before, you would understand my "internal GPS" was amazing. I had such an incredible sense of direction, and I thank my dad for those genes. I always was able to find my way around, even in an unfamiliar city. My friends looked to me to navigate new places when we were out adventuring.

Now, I get lost right in my own neighborhood.

Preparing to go to Washington, D.C. where I knew I would have to travel on the Metro/subway, my friend, Jill, helped me do my research so I would know exactly which line to take, and where to get on and off for my stops. I downloaded an app that gave me step-by-step instructions along the way. I understood that I needed to purchase a SmartTrip pass, yet when the time came to use the automated machine, I was baffled. There was a line of people behind me waiting to use the machine, so I pretended to do something, and then got out of line. I waited until the line went down, and then asked a young woman for assistance.

Once I got to my first subway line change, I was completely confused as to which side of the platform I needed to be on. I could read the sign, but was unable to process whether I needed to be on this side of the tracks or the other. I eventually asked someone for assistance, and got on the train going the correct direction. I have navigated Chicago many times in the past, as well as New York City's subway without any problems. But of course, this was before I had a TBI.

My "old life" is still so vivid in my memory, while my "new life" is completely different. I am easily frustrated by things that I used to be able to do effortlessly. I am slowly learning to embrace the "new normal" and understand my limits, but it's still hard. Especially when it comes to cognitive or memory issues that I know would have never stood in my way two years ago.

I have also come to understand that all of this has happened to me for reasons beyond my control. I have been called by the Universe to be a messenger, to educate the masses about TBI. While it is a leading cause of death in the United States, hardly anyone understands how devastating a concussion can truly be.

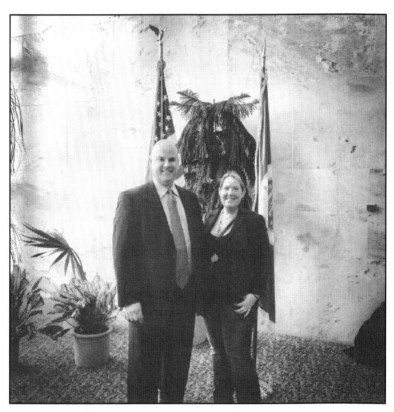

Paul Bosworth and me
in Washington, D.C.

Chapter 8

A Benefit for Brain Injury
in Breaux Bride, Louisiana

July 2015

I rolled into Breaux Bridge, Louisiana, during a rainstorm, with raindrops the size of gumballs falling so fast on my windshield that I can hardly see the car in front of me. It was over almost as quickly as it started. I have been told this is a typical mid-day shower in Cajun country, as daily "mini showers" roll in from the Gulf, lasting only a few minutes, but drenching the earth. The landscape is bright green, and lush, thanks to these showers.

I arrive at my hotel to be greeted by a lovely wreath on the front door. At first it appears they forgot to take down their Christmas decorations, but upon closer inspection I see they are covered in red crawfish and netting material, in honor of the Crawfish Festival celebrated here. I can't help but smile. It's the little things that make small towns so special.

April, a fellow survivor, my dog, Pixxie, and I, had loaded up the car and road tripped twelve hundred miles to Louisiana to support a cause near and dear to me: Traumatic Brain Injury. Paul Bosworth, my friend and a survivor, started BBQ4TBI several years ago in an effort to raise money and awareness for brain injury. The BBQ has taken on a life of its own, and now in their third year, has over thirty teams ready to take part in this state-sanctioned BBQ cook-off. Proceeds are to benefit the Brain Injury Alliance of Louisiana, and help bring awareness to TBI.

In addition to supporting the cause, I was selling my art and "awareness bracelets" at the BBQ. I am honored to have been a part of something so amazing. I had no idea how serious of a "sport" BBQ competitions are in the south. These folks take their BBQ very seriously, and their reputation is on the line. In addition to BBQ, we helped bring awareness to many others about TBI, which is the leading cause of death in Americans under the age of forty-five.

While living in Washington, D.C. Paul received a TBI after he choked on chicken fried rice. Alone in his kitchen, he passed out, hitting his head on the floor. When he came-to he still had food lodged in his throat, so he went into the bathroom in an attempt to remove it. The removal caused a tear in his throat, and he called his girlfriend to take him to the ER.

At first, the doctors were most concerned about the tear and bleeding. He was sent home, and told he had suffered a concussion. He went back to work, but as the days went on, it became apparent that he had suffered more brain damage than originally thought. He was having a hard time speaking, and would stutter frequently, and he was plagued with debilitating headaches. He had a difficult time reading and comprehending things. He eventually went to a neurologist, who told him he had post-concussion syndrome (PCS).

He quickly realized he wasn't going to be able to continue

working and went on short-term disability. He moved back home to Louisiana to be near family. Friends were slowly and gradually leaving him, they didn't understand this silent epidemic that he was living with.

After a few years, he knew he needed to do something to raise awareness as well as occupy his time. He put together the first BBQ in conjunction with a Jeep ride, and it was wildly successful. After doing it two years, the city of Breaux Bridge became involved, and it has evolved into a bigger and more exciting event. Organizing the BBQ gives Paul a sense of belonging, and his "work" as he is still on long-term disability. It also challenges his brain, and allows him to relearn skills that he had lost.

Upon our arrival in town, Paul graciously took us out to dinner at Prejeans for some authentic local cuisine. We had gator bites, boudin, shrimp fondeaux, effete, and so much more. For dessert we had sweet potato pecan pie, which was simply amazing. Pecan pie is one of my all-time favorites, and this took the cake (pun intended).

The BBQ started with us putting up our tent in a rain and windstorm. We almost lost the tent once to the wind, but we managed to get it up and get everything set up without getting soaked. Then the skies parted, and we had a beautiful, albeit steamy, afternoon. We had a few sales and met some great people. Most importantly, we helped support a great cause and raise awareness for TBI.

Paul has done something spectacular for brain injury awareness, and I want to extend a heartfelt "thank you" to Paul for all of his efforts. I know what kind of energy it takes to put on an event like this, and I also know it takes a toll on a brain injury.

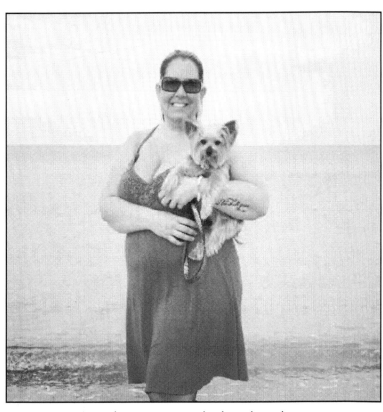

My Yorkie, Pixxie, at the beach with me

Chapter 9

Missing My Memory: Life with a TBI

August 2015

I used to have the most amazing memory. I had memorized friends' phone numbers, as well as all my credit card numbers, and my driver's license number. I could watch a movie once and recite all the one-liners on command. I could read an entire book in a day, or over the weekend (depending how long it was). I could multi-task like a mad woman, juggling five things at once. It was easy for me, and it was my normal.

After my fall, I had no idea the journey that I was about to begin, and the struggles that I would endure.

The most immediately apparent effects were short-term memory loss, cognitive functioning, and aphasia, which is not being able to recall words, or using the wrong word. I was originally told I had a severe concussion, and that most of my symptoms would resolve themselves in a few weeks.

All of a sudden it was eight weeks later, and I was still struggling. At that point, I had an MRI to rule out any major bleeding or damage. It fortunately came back clear, but that's not to say I didn't have minor tearing, which does not show up in imaging, and can cause long-term problems.

It was clear this was a traumatic brain injury, and there are no clear-cut "rules" on recovery. No two TBIs are the same. They have a lot of similar symptoms, however, the combination of those, and the length of time it takes to recover, can vary greatly.

I know survivors who had a mild TBI like I did, and have taken years to get better, while someone with a severe TBI, which means he was in a coma for an extended period of time, was almost fully recovered in a year or so. There is no magic formula, and no guarantees that you will ever completely recover.

Actually, most TBI survivors never make a full and complete recovery. They are left with some part of their brain impaired. We learn coping skills to help us: such as notebooks where we write down everything, GPS to help keep us from getting lost, calendars to keep track of appointments, and the like. However, even with all the coping mechanisms in the world, there is no substitute for the way it was before. I am now the sticky note queen.

Adapting to your "new normal" is incredibly frustrating. Especially when the "old you" is so vivid in your long-term memory. You know how you used to function, and you expect that part of you to come back at the snap of your fingers. But it doesn't. It takes time—lots of time. And the more time that passes, the more frustrating it becomes.

Julia Potocnjak-Overn from Tyler, Texas, sustained her TBI after a car accident two years ago. She sums up her memory:

"My memory is kind of like a garbled sentence. Bits and

pieces here and there, but no clear thoughts. Lots of half thoughts, or thoughts that disappear into the abyss. I get frustrated by having a difficult time remembering daily tasks, questions, or even trying to find the right word."

Heather L. George from New Brighton, Minnesota, suffered two TBIs within two years of each other, in 2012 and 2014. She struggles with memory issues like I do, and has found a useful coping skill:

"I used to have a very "tape-recorder-quality" memory, now I expend a lot of brain energy trying to make sure that I haven't forgotten something, or panicking, and literally losing sleep because I fear that I may have forgotten something.

"When I pass the stove on my way to let the dog outside, I set the stove timer so that it reminds me to let him in. I use the stove timer a lot to remind me of things such as: when the oven should be done preheating, when I should check water to see if it is boiling, when I should tend to items that are soaking, etc. It works as long as I remember why I have set it. If I don't, it at least makes for an amusing treasure hunt."

Kara Harkins from Lexington, Kentucky, suffered a TBI in 2012 after a car pulled out in front of hers. She has no memory of the accident, and presently suffers from memory issues:

"I have short-term memory issues. Not tragic like so many stories I see and read, but because it is so invisible, very few people understand or even try. I get extremely frustrated trying to learn new things. I can't keep up with notebooks because I loose them, or don't remember what the notes mean. I survive on lots of reminders in my smartphone. My issues are diagnosed as permanent, and I am on disability. My ten-year-old daughter is my biggest reason for getting up each day, and provides a great source to help me recall things, and she also reminds me of things."

I think the fact that we can still remember who we were before the injury makes it even more frustrating for us. Even with coping skills to help us in the moment, we are forever reminded of who we once were.

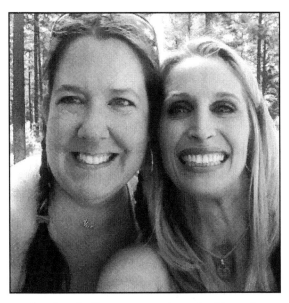

Stephanie Freeman and me in Georgia

Chapter 10

Ten Ways You Can Help
a Loved One Cope With a TBI

August 2015

In a recent conversation with my fellow TBI survivors, we were discussing ways that people can reach out and help us. The first few months after a concussion or traumatic brain injury are critical. When I look back at my first six months, I can see how completely dazed and confused I was.

However, the recovery from a TBI can last from months to years. Every single brain injury is unique, and will take different recovery times, and also present different symptoms, depending on where the brain was injured. There is no "magic formula," and I know of those with diagnosed "severe" TBI who fully recovered in a few years, while others with a "mild" TBI are still recovering many years later.

A TBI is much like a fingerprint or snowflake—no two are alike.

In addition, many "outsiders" have no idea what kind of hell we are going through. They hear the word "concussion," and think it's not big deal. Or they hear the term, "traumatic brain injury," and can only imagine the most severe situations—think coma, bedridden, not able to speak or walk—and figure if we're walking and talking, then we must be doing "OK." Neither of these scenarios is correct, and I beg of you to try to understand what we're going through. At the very least, I offer you some suggestions on how to help us cope with this stressful and frustrating time of our life.

1. Don't ask us what we need. We may not actually know "what" we need. Or we may feel embarrassed, and don't want to be a burden or seem needy. Don't ask us if we'd like you to come over. We'll likely say no, but in truth, mean yes. Show up at our door with open arms.

2. Bring over a meal (or three). We are likely suffering from a great deal of fatigue, headaches, and cognitive problems. We might not have the ability to cook for ourselves, or even go to the grocery store to buy the bare necessities. I couldn't figure out how to use my microwave or oven. A warm, home-cooked meal would have been greatly appreciated.

3. Bring us groceries or basic household supplies. As much as we won't admit it, our finances are going to be really, really tight. Going to the grocery store might actually be a financial burden as much as it is a physical one. No one wants to admit when they're struggling, and if you show up with some milk, toilet paper, and chocolate chip cookies, it will definitely bring joy and relief.

4. Offer to clean our house. Many of us suffer with vertigo, fatigue, and likely we have physical injuries from our accident. Simple tasks like taking out the garbage, doing laundry, and vacuuming can be daunting. Don't judge the condition of our home, and don't make us feel like we are doing a poor job of house keeping, simply enter our home and start doing it for us. Take it a step further, and make us a glass of ice water, tuck us into bed for a nap, and clean away while we rest.

5. Offer to drive us to our doctor appointments. I was fortunate that I was able to drive after my accident, but many are not. I also encourage you to ask if we'd like you to sit in on the appointment. I went to all my appointments alone, and as I look back, I realize how little I remember. It would have been nice to have someone along to help advocate for my health, and to be able to explain to the doctor what she is observing of my daily behavior, and how it may be altered from my "normal.

6. Get us out of the house. Before you kidnap your loved one and take her on an adventure, make sure you ask if she is feeling up to it. If it is an adventure that comes with some monetary costs, make it clear that you are buying—remember how I mentioned that finances may be extremely tight. Keep in mind that they may be sensitive to light, sounds, crowds, etc., and plan something accordingly. A trip to a flower garden (remind her to bring her sunglasses),

or to a spa for a pedicure, might be lovely options. Or you can ask her what she'd like to do, but be prepared that she might not be able to articulate a clear plan. Be prepared to plan it all out.

7. Bring this person flowers. I know that's totally cliché, but beautiful flowers can brighten up anyone's day.

8. Send a card or care package. If you don't live nearby, sending a card with a note saying you're thinking of them will mean so very much. Knowing you are in someone's thoughts can go a long way in recovery. If you're feeling generous, you may also include a gift card to a local grocery or Target store.

9. Show up with a movie and a book. Ask if we would prefer to watch a movie, or have you read to us. Everyone's TBI is going to be different. Some can't handle watching a movie or hearing the sounds, and many can't read well. So offering to read a book might make our day. If neither seem appealing to us at the time, snuggle up with us on the couch under a comfy blanket, and simply be there for us. Sometimes sitting in silence with a loved one can truly make a person's day.

10. Watch our kids for a few hours. Or better yet, take the children overnight. Being a parent with TBI must be overwhelming and exhausting. Knowing that our children are in good hands will give us comfort and allow us to rest and recharge for a few hours. Rest is so important in the recovery process.

Also know that we are in this for the long haul. We will still be struggling with the lasting effects of our injury for months, if not years, after the accident. Don't put pressure on your loved one that he "should" be feeling better. I am eighteen months out, and still suffer a great deal of fatigue and cognitive deficits, as well as regular headaches.

Be aware that we tend to be incredibly emotional after a head injury, or possibly even aggressive. Be prepared that your generosity will elicit many emotions, some will cry, some will laugh, and some might possibly get angry with you. Don't take any of it personally. We are dealing with a very difficult injury, not to mention a complete change in our personality. Realize you are doing the best you can for us, and that we appreciate you, no matter how we may react.

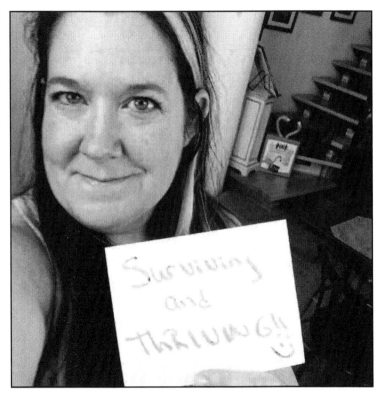

This photo of me was featured in a Cristabelle Braden music video for her song, "Hope Survives."

Chapter 11

Anxiety, Depression, and
Traumatic Brain Injury

October 2015

Living with a traumatic brain injury can be a very lonely, painful place. It's a place that is often misunderstood, and a place that no one is talking about.

When I first fell on a patch of ice nineteen months ago, I had no idea the journey that laid ahead—the ups and downs—and the feeling of moving backwards instead of forward. Also, I feel isolated—that no one understands, or even believes, what I'm going through.

My original diagnosis was that I had a severe concussion. I was told that my symptoms should get better in a few weeks, and that extreme emotions are typical. I remember crying while watching anything on television, even comedy. I had an overwhelming sense of sadness, for no apparent reason, *all the time.*

I rarely wanted to leave the house, as public places were too loud and over-stimulating. In the rare instance that I did go out with friends, I would have this feeling in the pit of my stomach that I couldn't figure out. I would have a hard time breathing, and would be fighting back tears most of the time. I usually ended up leaving early with an excuse that I was getting a headache—although that was often the truth.

About ten months after my fall, my symptoms were not getting any better, and some were actually getting worse, or new ones were appearing. Later I found out this was typical. I started slipping deeper into depression, thinking I was never going to get better. I couldn't handle the intense pain and fatigue that were a constant in my new world. I began having a lot of fear related to falling again, or hurting myself in general. I was over protective of my body. Often I would not leave my house, all the while reasoning in my head that I could not get hurt again if I didn't go near the icy sidewalks.

I had never suffered from anxiety before my fall, other than the standard "butterflies in the stomach" feeling the night before a big presentation or other event. This feeling now building inside me was unfamiliar, and I truly didn't know what was happening to me, or how to control it.

I had dislocated my sternum in the fall, and had a lot of soreness in my chest. I didn't give the pain much thought, until it started getting worse, and it was coupled with a rapid heart rate and sweaty palms. I felt like my throat was closing, and I couldn't breathe. All I wanted to do was scream as tears started rolling down my cheeks.

Thankfully my good friend recognized what was happening. She was pretty sure I was having an *anxiety attack*. She told me to go ahead and scream because it would make me feel better. Words started coming out of my mouth from somewhere deep within my body. I heard myself saying things like, "I am so sick of feeling like this." "I want to get better…. to feel normal again." "I can't handle all this pain." "All of this pain and fatigue is too much."

After the anxiety attack, I was completely drained of all energy and emotion. I spent the next few weeks walking around in a zombie-like manner, and I barely had enough energy to walk, let alone talk to someone. I spent most of my time in bed, or staring blankly at the television screen.

Now that I am aware of what that feeling was, I am better able to manage it. However, at times it still gets a grip on me, and will paralyze me to the core with fear. I have found meditation and yoga help ease the rising feeling in my chest, and draw my attention to my breath instead of the fear. Anxiety is a seriously scary thing that you truly have no control over. I am surprised what sets it off, and of course, it happens when I am least expecting it. Other times, like when we got our first snowy-ice mixture the following winter, it makes sense to me.

Christi Smith from Sturgis, Michigan, suffered a TBI in 2009 after she fell out of a moving golf cart. She says:

"My anxiety, depression and PTSD affect me every day. Some days I have bursts of anger, and others I'm extremely emotional and cry about most things. I'm always anxious about everything."

Julie Nowak from Toronto, Ontario, Canada suffred a TBI in 2014 from a biking accident. She says:

"We live in an 'able-ist' world that does not know how to deal with mental health. When I tell people about my anxiety, I am told to stop worrying. We don't tell some-one in a wheelchair to walk, so why would you tell an anxious person to stop being anxious? We need to have more empathy, and we need people who will be with us during our struggles, and love us regardless, rather than tell us to change. Large, loud groups of people trigger my social anxiety, and I often cannot be in these spaces. Yet if I want to socialize with my peers who are in their twenties and thirties, these group settings are typically my only options. Thus, I am forced to choose between anxiety and loneliness."

Anxiety and depression tend to go hand in hand, and are extremely common for those with TBI and chronic pain. I am fortunate to have found a great therapist who is helping me work though my fears, and he is also teaching me how to get a better grip on them.

I strongly urge anyone who is suffering to seek the help and guidance of a therapist. There is no need to torture yourself by going through these feelings alone. There truly is light at the end of the tunnel, and when we are stuck in a dark place, it is challenging to see that.

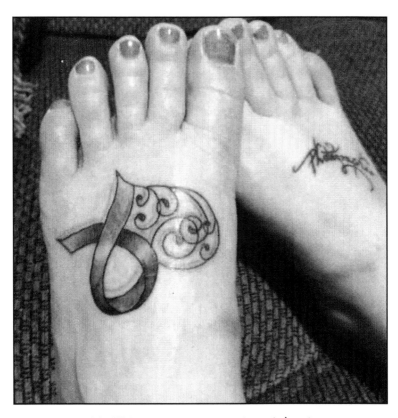

My TBI awareness tattoo (yes, it hurt)

Chapter 12

Miss America Contestant is a
Voice for Traumatic Brain Injury

September 2015

I had the pleasure of chatting with Ali Wallace, currently Miss Oregon. Early September 2015, she will head to Atlantic City to compete in the Miss America Pageant. Ali is a beautiful, smart, young woman who also happens to have an invisible injury that she struggles with every day—a traumatic brain injury.

In her freshman year of high school, she made the varsity cheer team. This was a very distinct honor not given to many freshmen. She felt a bit of pressure to keep up with the other girls on her team, and would practice her tumbling skills outside of practice.

One afternoon, she was at the dance studio working on her round-off back tuck. She wasn't comfortable with this move yet, and she became nervous in the middle of her flip, resulting in her falling to the floor. She landed half on the mat and half on the hardwood floor, with the back of her head/upper neck hitting first. Her mom saw it happen, and rushed over to assist her.

Ali immediately knew that something wasn't quite right.

She had completely lost vision in her left eye, and had de-
creased vision in her right. She was seeing stars and feeling woozy.
Her mom called the nurse line to see if they should bring her in
to see a doctor, and was assured that she should be fine—and to
just go home and rest. In fact, Mom was told not to bother bring-
ing Ali in to the clinic.

Her accident occurred in 2009, a time when concussions were
"no big deal," a time when athletes were sent back on the field to
play, and a time when doctors didn't understand that there might
be long-term lasting effects. Even today, many people can misun-
derstand concussions, including medical professionals.

While awareness is growing as NFL players come forward and
tell their stories, this isn't enough. When the average person hears
the word "concussion," he or she might think *it's no big deal.* When
people hear the words "traumatic brain injury," they imagine the
worst-case scenarios—people who are in a coma or confined to a
wheelchair. This simply isn't the case, as one can see when looking
at Miss Oregon.

More survivors of concussions need to step forward and shed
light on the issue, which is exactly what Ali is doing. She is using
her platform at the Miss America competition to bring a face and
a voice to this debilitating injury.

The day after her accident, Ali's entire body ached all over.
Light hurt her eyes, sounds made her head throb, it hurt to read,
and she was feeling dizzy and nauseous. Her mom once again
called the nurse line, and finally Ali was instructed to go see her
doctor.

As soon as her primary doctor saw her, he knew something
wasn't right. He ordered a brain scan, which showed some minor

bleeding on her brain. While it didn't require surgery, Ali was told she had suffered a traumatic brain injury. She was instructed to stay home from school for a month to rest and recover.

Ali said, "When I took a month off of school, there was a combination of jealousy, and those who thought I was just trying to get out of going to school. You can't see a concussion, it's not like a broken arm where you can see it's broken."

At her follow-up appointment, she wasn't able to see her regular doctor. This doctor now told her "If you can put on your makeup, then you are fine." His statement stunned both Ali and her mom.

Sadly, this is an all-too-often generalization: If you look fine, can talk and walk, then you must be okay. It is extremely frustrating to survivors, and can be quite disheartening.

Ali continued with her follow-up appointments, seeing her regular doctor. She was still feeling dizzy and nauseous, and was told that it could take about a year to get back to feeling normal. While her friends were out having fun, she spent all of her summer break resting in a dark, quiet room, trying to give her brain adequate time to heal and recover.

"You're brain controls your entire body. If your brain is injured, things don't work correctly," Ali commented.

After missing an entire year of cheer team, her doctor cleared her to return. Ali shared that mentally she was never able to do tumbles again, as she always had a small fear in the pit of her stomach. She didn't want to risk another bad landing, and injure herself more. Regardless of her fears, she put her best effort into the cheer team, and continued to thrive during her last two years of high school.

Six years later, Ali continues to struggle with the aftereffects of her TBI.

Ali has frequent headaches, and lacks depth perception in her left eye, which causes her to sometimes run into doorways or other objects that are on her left side. She has a lot of balance issues, which has put a damper on her dancing. She struggles with aphasia (being able to recall words), and has mastered the art of redirecting her sentence, using a different word. She also gets lost while driving, often having to pull over and try to figure out where she was headed by looking at her calendar.

Her biggest fear in the Miss America competition is being perceived as not being intelligent, especially when she can't come up with a word quickly enough. "It's embarrassing to be stuck in the middle of a sentence, and not be able to think of the right word."

Those who have never struggled with a TBI have no idea how frustrating aphasia can be, and outsiders who see a very pretty face sometimes make unfair assumptions and judgments.

Ali uses lots of lists to cope with her memory problems, spending time each night before bed writing down what she needs to do the next day. She continues to have sensitivity to light and sound, and struggles to remember people's names. Overall she is doing great, and will be attending Portland State next summer to finish her BA degree. She plans to pursue a Masters of Film degree from the University of Southern California.

When she selected to talk about TBI as her platform, she wanted to bring awareness to a topic that nobody is talking about. She has personal, first-hand experience with it, and is a cause that she wants to continue to shed light on and support.

Her biggest message she wants to bring the world is this: "I want people to understand how serious TBI is. When the conversations of brain injuries come up, I want it to be general knowledge of how serious and complex the injury is. No two brains heal alike, and it's not like a bone where the standard recovery time is 4–6 weeks. The minimum recovery time for a very mild concussion is three months. Unfortunately, there is no formula to know when you'll recover or heal."

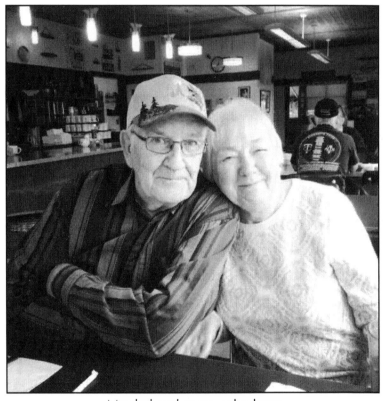

My dad and mom, who have
supported me throughout my recovery

Chapter 13

How Essential Oils Helped Me Cope
With a Traumatic Brain Injury

August 2015

Right before my fall, I had started using essential oils, and having these oils on hand was the biggest blessing. They helped me cope with my traumatic brain injury, along with the physical injuries I sustained, which included whiplash, torn muscles, stretched ligaments, and a dislocated sternum and ribcage.

What I am about to share with you is my own personal experience with essential oils. Not everyone will have the exact same results, and *not all oils are created equally.*

The oils sold at health food stores and co-ops are *not* 100 percent therapeutic grade oils, meaning that you don't know what else has been added to them. They may state on the label that they indeed are therapeutic grade or 100 percent pure, because there is zero regulation on essential oils. But if you look closely, the label will say things like "external use only" and "dilute properly." These are red flags that the oil in that bottle is not 100 percent, and it has likely been cut with other oils or chemicals. Be sure to do your research before using an oil—and never, ever ingest an oil if you unsure whether it is 100 percent therapeutic grade.

You will notice that with many of the oils I use a cool mist diffuser, which diffuses the oils into the air for an aromatic benefit. I have found that my skin allows me to put most oils directly onto it; however, it is recommended that you use *a carrier oil* such as coconut, almond, or even vegetable oil if you have nothing else. One drop of essential oil and one drop of carrier oil, and you're set to go.

Below is a list of my symptoms, and the oils I used to treat them:

- Brain fog: I diffuse a few drops of *cedarwood* at night while I sleep. If I am traveling, I will put a few drops on the back of my neck and wrists. I notice a huge difference in clarity when I wake up after a night of inhaling diffused cedarwood.

- Muscle pain: I use an all natural pain-relieving gel called *Arnica*, which you can find at most health food stores or coops. I rub it into my sore spots with a few drops of *peppermint*. I also made a roller ball of this to roll directly onto the spot to have along when I'm on the go.

- Headaches: *Peppermint* minimizes my headaches. I apply a few drops to the base of my neck, temples, or scalp, whatever is hurting me at the moment. I have made a roller ball of peppermint as well for easy application. I *always* have peppermint with me, in my purse, in my suitcase, in my laptop case, everywhere. This is my number one go-to oil for so many things. I truly never leave home without it.

- Ligaments: I stretched a few ligaments in my neck, and they are especially challenging to recover. I have found *lemongrass* to be very helpful in encouraging them back to their original plasticity. I use this in combination with peppermint and Arnica when applying to my neck in the morning and evening.

- Sleep: I diffuse *vertiver* at bedtime, and will combine with *cedarwood* if I am foggy. When traveling, I will put it directly on my writs and the front of my throat. It has a warm, smoky smell, and puts me right to sleep. (Note: I also take Melatonin supplements to aid in sleep.)

- Immune support: I put one drop of *lemon* in my glass water bottle every day, and haven't had even a sniffle in over a year. I also use *thieves* (a blend) for extra support when going out to crowded places, or when I know I will be around small children because they are such effective "germ carriers." For thieves, I will put a drop on the bottom of my foot after a hot bath or shower, and I will also rub a drop inside my nose. (Note: this will sting the first few times you do it.) I make sure I am rubbing it into the membranes, and not snorting it up my nose.

- Relaxation: Whenever I take a bath, which is about three times a week, I add three drops of *lavender* to my water. It not only is relaxing, it also softens your skin, smells great, and keeps you from drying out in the winter months. Be careful getting in and out because your tub can be slippery when using oil. Also, don't bother with bubble bath because the oils will keep it from making bubbles. I will also use a drop with a quarter-size amount of coconut oil that I purchase at any grocery store, and rub into my skin. This leaves your skin so soft and radiant, and will smell divine. If you are sore, I also suggest adding Epsom salts to your bath as it helps draw out the toxins from your muscles. I noticed a *lot* of relief when doing this.

- Anxiety: My drug of choice for anxiety and panic attacks is an essential oil: a blend called *transformation*. This one is a bit spendy, but it works so amazing for me, and is way cheaper than paying for prescriptions. A bottle has lasted me a year, so it was money well spent. All I have to do is smell the bottle, and I am immediately calmed. I will wear a few drops on my throat and wrists if I am going out and feel anxious.

- Neck and sternum: I had a dislocated sternum, and my C4 was pushed into C5. For this I used *valor*, which is commonly referred to as "chiropractor in a bottle." I apply a drop or two in each area, and I apply on my neck before applying my lemongrass and peppermint mixture.

- Mood: I will inhale *lemon, or orange,* or diffuse them. I have found diffusing lemon greatly lifts my mood almost immediately if I am feeling "blah."

- Dizzy and balance: I put a drop of *ginger* behind each ear. For a more immediate result, I will also sniff it as

I am applying it.

- Acid reflux: I use a drop of *peppermint* and rub into the area from my stomach up through my esophagus. I notice relief almost immediately.

- Fatigue: Smelling *peppermint* (or diffusing it) will give me a pick-me-up if I am feeling fatigued. Also, a small drop on my tongue can help me perk up as well, plus you get the added fresh-breath bonus. You can also rub a drop on your chest or neck for a longer lasting effect.

I strongly suggest you consult with someone well versed in essential oils before beginning a regimen.

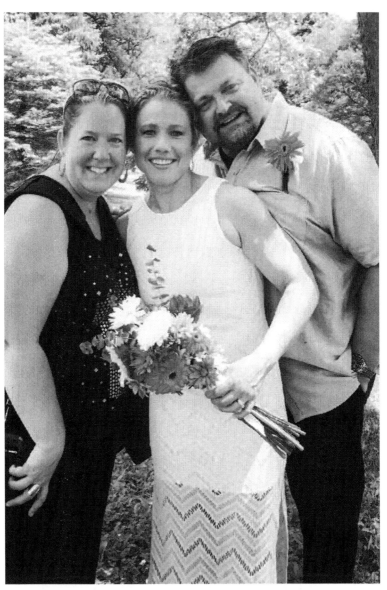

With my trainer, Belinda, and my doctor,
Fred Clary, at their wedding. Both have
been instrumental in my recovery

Chapter 14

A Ready-to-Send Care Package
for Traumatic Brain Injury

July 2015

Recently I partnered with Grace Quantock, one of my beautiful friends from the United Kingdom, and founder of Healing Boxes. She began Healing Boxes in 2012 after a friend was in a car accident, and was recovering in the hospital.

Grace said,

"At the time I was bedbound. Although I could not visit, I wanted to do something for my friend. I felt helpless in that moment, and it was awful. I was too far away to visit, and felt there was little I could do, until I realized I could send my support, in a healing, heartwarming box of cheer. It sounded so simple, so obvious. But as I began to search for the right gift, I was utterly disheartened by what little was available and appropriate. A card and flowers was just not enough.

"Being homebound and living with a chronic illness myself, I knew exactly what was needed. So I searched and packaged up a variety of lovingly items that my dear friend would enjoy, and be able to use. The very first Healing Box was born."

Healing Boxes became more than a business, it became a mission. Grace wanted to spread comfort, joy, passion, and love to every person in need. She assembled a board of fantastic people who were passionate about helping others, and formally made Healing Boxes a "Community Interest Company" (CIC). A CIC is a UK-based type of company that is specifically designed to use their profits and assets for the public good and the benefit of the community. Basically, it's a business and charity all rolled into one neat little package, or in her case, a box.

Grace is currently thriving while living with an often-debilitating illness. She knows firsthand the emotional and physical roller coaster that accompanies diagnosis and life struggle. This is exactly why I knew Grace was the perfect person to partner with for a TBI Healing Box. Of course, I knew exactly what it was like. You feel alone, isolated, scared, emotional, and mostly, you just want someone to reach out to you with love and compassion.

The TBI Healing Box is filled with items Grace and I lovingly selected specifically for individuals dealing with traumatic brain injury or post-concussion syndrome. All of the items are handmade in the UK, and include:

- Ear plugs, to help keep distracting and overwhelming noises to a minimum.
- Eye mask, to help with light sensitivity.
- Ice pack, to help with sore muscles, as well as headaches.
- Meditation CD, specifically designed to help with sleep.

- Palm stone, as a reminder of the love and support that was sent your way.
- Teapigs Tea bags, for a comforting and soothing cup of tea.
- Wellness Journal, to journal your recovery, keep track of to-do items, and more.
- Hand-written note from the sender to encourage you on your journey to recovery.

All of this is lovingly packaged in Wales, UK and delivered to the door of your loved one. Imagine the gratitude this person will feel, knowing someone has thought enough to send this Healing Box, specific to the invisible injury that he is currently feeling overwhelmed and struggling with.

This Healing Box is designed for a loved one you care about, who has either recently suffered a concussion or brain injury, or is still continuing to recover from one because recovery can take years. Consider sending one if you have a loved one you care about, but feel you:

- Want to do something for them but don't know what to do.
- Are scared and frustrated.
- Feel out of your league on the scope of their injury.
- Don't understand their injury.
- Don't live nearby to help or visit, or
- Want to help, but don't know how.

I know first-hand the struggle, and these are the exact items I have used to help me with my recovery. It is hard to know what to do for someone when it's an injury that's invisible—one you cannot see or understand. By sending them a beautiful box full of useful items, designed just for what they are dealing with, you will show them just how much you care.

Best of all, you are not only helping a loved one suffering with TBI, you are also helping to support a community with the purchase of a Healing Box. For more information, please visit: www.healing-boxes.com/tbi

Note: These convenient-to-order Healing Boxes are available for about $50, including shipping to the anyone in the U.S.—and will be worth so much to that special person receiving it.

Part Two:

Finding the Road Back to Normal

Part Two is a series of short blog posts from my website, intending to inspire, and were written when I turned the corner in my own recovery.

Triumphant

by Amy Zellmer

I am floating
   weightless
I am spinning
   spiraling
Images are blurry
   fuzzy
Sound is echoing
   ringing
Nothing is certain
   confused
I have fallen
   crumpled
I am alive
   triumphant
The words are lost
   vanished
The thoughts are incomplete
   fragmented
Time is meaningless
   fleeting
Energy is low
   exhausted
I am alive
   triumphant

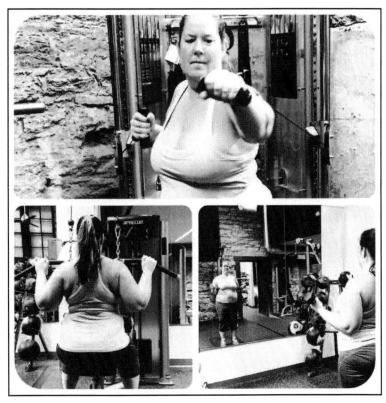

My trainer has me on a weight-training path to recovery

Chapter 15

Gratitude

September 2015

I've had something on my mind for a while, and I finally feel the need to write about it. In the beginning, I rarely talked about my injuries, as I had been made to feel ashamed by people I had considered friends because they didn't understand—and thought I was faking things. Their treatment left me horribly depressed, as I felt I had no one to turn to during this incredibly frightening time of my life. I had no idea how to use my microwave, I thought Bill Clinton was still President, and I had to look at my calendar every fifteen minutes to make sure I wasn't missing an appointment because I couldn't remember beyond that limited timeframe. I can't even begin to describe how scary the situation was to me, especially living alone. I had severe dizziness, body aches from the physical injuries, and I couldn't stand up straight for over a year, and the fatigue was debilitating, causing me to sleep twelve to fourteen hours at night, plus one or two naps during the day.

At my one-year mark, I became *beyond frustrated*. I had actually considered taking my life because I couldn't deal with it anymore—I didn't think I was ever going to recover from my TBI. But alas, I am a total and complete wuss, and knew I could never go thru with it. So I took to writing as my therapy. I can't tell you how thankful I am that 1) I didn't actually jump, and 2) I had the courage to submit my story to *The Huffington Post*.

My story has been read by literally tens of thousands of people. I have made friends from all over the world, brought together by TBI. I have helped *so many others* cope with their TBI and to understand that what they're dealing with is "normal," and they are most definitely not alone in this journey— all because I had the courage to put into words exactly how I felt. Words are powerful because they allow others a portal into your heart and soul.

Photographer friends and Facebook friends have reached out to me because a client or a friend of theirs has suffered a concussion/TBI, and they wanted to connect me with that person. It is absolutely amazing to me how writing one little blog post about little ol' me has turned into something that was special. Survivors so badly needed somewhere to turn, a place where they could chat with others dealing with the same issues.

It's been a pretty bumpy ride, but one that I am so incredibly thankful to be on. I knew the instant I fell that there was a bigger reason. At the time I had no idea what that reason would be, and I still don't know where exactly it is going to take me. But I can tell you that I am thankful *for you*. If you are reading this, then you have a special place in my heart, and I appreciate you. I am honored to be a part of your life, and wish you the very best in your recovery (or the recovery of your loved one). Thanks for taking this journey with me.

#TBIawareness #SurvivorsROCK #TBI

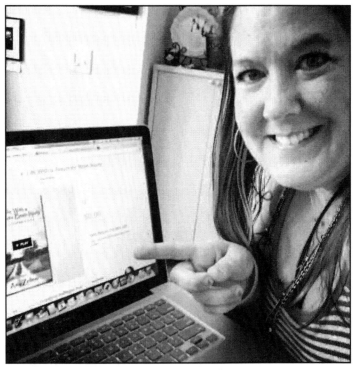

This is me on the day I launched
my Kickstarter campaign

Chapter 16

Musing

September 2015

I am often asked where I get my energy and motivation to continue writing about traumatic brain injury on *The Huffington Post*, or deciding to publish my book on the subject. I have received countless emails similar to this one from a mother in Kansas City, Missouri. *This is what inspires me to keep going.*

"Hi Amy,

I read your Life with a Traumatic Brain Injury article last night. I cried my way through it.

My 14-year-old daughter fell off the top of my husband's truck eight months ago trying to take a picture of the sunset. She loves photography and sunsets. She was home alone with her younger sister at the time, and called me to tell me how pretty the sunset was. She told me she was going to take a picture. Had she mentioned that she was going to climb on top of a truck to take that picture, things might be different than they are today.

I sent her your article, and she came to me in tears,

telling me she could have written it—that everything you wrote, she feels. That she doesn't even like telling people anymore what happened, but feels judged when it takes her a bit of time to count out money for her chai. The simple tasks are no longer simple. I, as a mom, feel helpless.

But you have helped us both. She is not alone. Others are out there that know how she feels. She is one determined, bright girl.

THANK you for opening up! Thank you, thank you, thank you!!"

Daily I receive emails and Facebook messages from survivors around the world telling me how much my writing has meant to them, as well as The TBI Tribe Facebook group. When I am feeling low, or fatigued, all I have to do is look at these words. They are what keep me going.

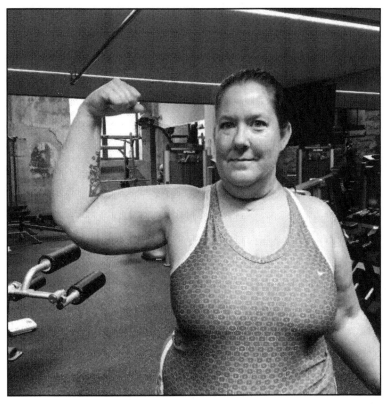

Here I am in the workout room,
showing off my new muscles

Chapter 17

Strength in Recovery

October 2015

My hope is that my recovery progress can help at least one other person begin gaining back his or her strength, and take back control over her/his life.

I am nineteen months post TBI, and when I fell, I suffered severe whiplash, torn muscles in my neck, shoulder, and chest, and dislocated my sternum by about *two inches*. My torso was completely twisted, and I couldn't stand up straight for over a year.

We tried integrating light weight training into my routine several times, but it kept flaring up that darn whiplashed muscle, so we would back off. I started doing very gentle yoga about three months ago. The doctors kept telling me that activity is the best way to overcome vertigo, which seemed counter intuitive, and yoga seemed the best place to start, as I could completely control which moves I did.

Within about two months, I started noticing my vertigo wasn't as severe, and my neck muscles were relaxing. I was also starting to see definition in my shoulders and chest again, and the inflammation had seemed to settle down. We didn't want to push too hard, so I just started adding cardio into my routine at that point.

This past week we added very light weight resistance into my workout. The first day, my neck got pretty angry, but I iced it, which relieved it. The neck is still being finicky, but I am powering through it. It isn't unbearable like the whiplash injury was, although it may take me out for a day if it gets really bad and triggers a headache. *Ice is my best friend.*

My dear friend and fellow survivor, Stephanie Freeman from Georgia, has been an inspiration to watch. She was in a car accident in 1993, which resulted in her being in a coma for two months. She was told she'd never be able to walk again, or have children. Here she is twenty-two years later; she has a son and is running marathons on a regular basis. She told me:

> "I have used activity to overcome anxiety and depression for many years, and found we can allow action to be an excellent and healthy therapy for our troubles. The greatest advice I can give is to get active. Our body has intelligent ways of healing itself, including our beautiful brains."

I hope that you read this, and become inspired to pull out the yoga mat and do some light stretches, or maybe go for a longer walk than usual, or maybe you're even ready to grab some weights. Whatever it is, listen to your body because it will tell you what it can and can't do. But the best thing you can do for your TBI is to get up and get moving—and have ice packs waiting in the wings. Also remember to keep hydrated because our brains love water, and stay away from drugs and alcohol as they impair our brain's ability to heal.

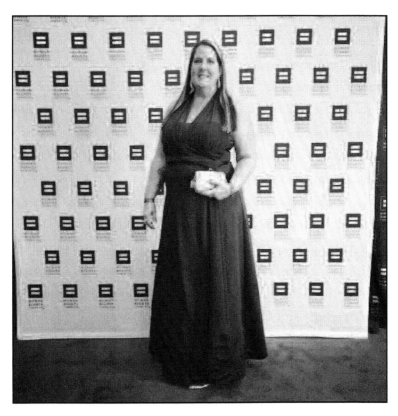

All dressed up at the Human Rights
Campaign gala in Minneapolis

Chapter 18

I Survived a Gala

September 2015

On a Saturday night in September I attended the Human Rights Campaign "red carpet gala" in Minneapolis. It was the first "big" outing I've attended in the past nineteen months. I managed to walk 17,000 steps that night, doing so in heels, and interacted with people for about three hours. I listened to speakers/presenters for about an hour during dinner. In the moment, I actually felt pretty good, and was proud of my body and brain for doing so well.

Then on Sunday, I slept pretty much all day, still felt miserable the next day, and I was still feeling the effects a day later. It's unreal how what many people take for granted as a simple outing, puts us into a tailspin for days. I popped ibuprofen, iced my neck, and drank lots of water in an attempt to recover.

TBI isn't something that you can "just recover" from— it takes years, and even then you may never make a full recovery. Our brains are easily over stimulated and can shut down on us after too much. Everyone has different symptoms and reacts to situations differently, as no two brain injuries are alike. #TBI #awareness

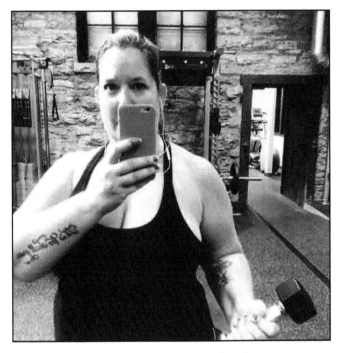

Seeing changes in my body after just
three weeks in the weight room

Chapter 19

Recovery is an Attitude

October 2015

They say a picture is worth a thousand words…

It's been nineteen months since I fell on a patch of ice, landing full-force on the back of my skull. I suffered a traumatic brain injury plus whiplash, torn muscles in my neck, shoulder and chest, and I also dislocated my sternum.

What this photo doesn't show is how I wasn't able to do any exercise, even mild, for the first year. Just walking around the grocery store was enough to leave my energy spent for the rest of the day, and I still had to carry the bags of groceries into the house.

I am not exaggerating when I tell you that I lived pretty much in my bed or on the couch for over a year. I would schedule photography sessions a few times a week because I had bills to pay, and that's my ONLY form of income. However, I would pay the price for two days, and needed to ice my aching neck, and pop ibuprofen like it was candy. Yay to the fact that I've since quit this pill habit.

Even just six months ago, I couldn't properly stand up

straight, let alone do strength training. And let's not forget about the horrible vertigo and balance issues that came with the TBI. But I finally decided that *enough is enough*. It was time to do something—anything, so I started doing yoga for about ten to fifteen minutes a day.

At first it was *really hard*. I could do only very basic, simple stretching yoga poses, and would hold onto a chair for any standing poses so I didn't lose my balance. But *it helped*, and started me on a path to gaining back my strength and endurance.

And now look at me. I am working with a fabulous trainer, and we are using weights and resistance to get my body back to pre-injury status. It feels so good to be able to walk standing fully upright, and have the strength to carry my groceries into the house. I feel absolutely amazing, and my physical symptoms are subsiding, but the neurological ones are still present.

I know it seems impossible when you're in the darkest days after a TBI. I've been there. But when you finally start to step out of it and say, "Screw you, TBI," you take back control of your life. If I can do this, *I know you can, too*.

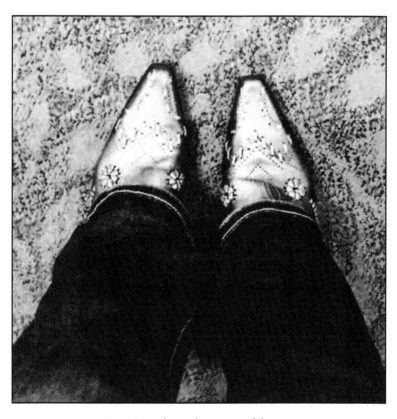

Exciting day when I could wear
heels for the first time since I fell

Chapter 20

The Power of Shoes

October 2015

Shoes.

While you may look at this photo and find it rather irrelevant, you do not understand its significance.

They look like cute shoes that I would have worn every day in my "old" life. Cute. Comfy. My go-to pair.

But up until just a few weeks ago, I never would have ventured out in shoes with heels. While they are relatively low, wide heels, nonetheless they are heels.

For the past 20 months, I have been living inside a life that didn't feel like my own. My TBI left me foggy, slow to think, and with impaired working memory. I have felt like a complete stranger, all alone in this bizarre world.

No one could tell me how long I'd feel this way, if I would ever return to "normal."

Shoes.

Today I wore these shoes.

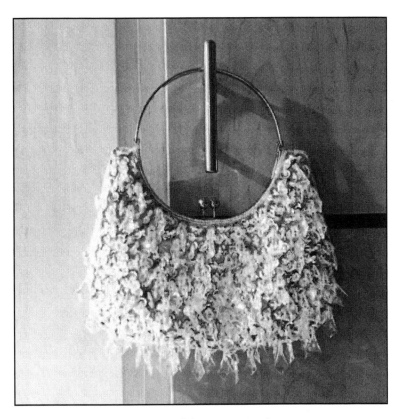

My Carrie Bradshaw-inspired purse

Chapter 21

The Significance of a Purse

October 2015

This afternoon I submitted my manuscript to my editor. It's *almost done*! To celebrate, a friend and I went out to dinner and shopping. I splurged and bought this purse.

The purse looks like something Carrie Bradshaw would own in "Sex and the City." Here's the significance is this: About three months ago I decided to watch my "Sex and the City" full-series DVD collection—for the third time. Only this time, I had zero memory of having seen any of the episodes. This was TBI memory loss at its finest.

Fast forward to the scene where a publisher approaches Carrie with the idea to turn her column into a book. I had an ah-ha moment. I could turn my *Huffington Post* articles into a book.

I was on a mission. I set a goal. I set a date for my book release. And now here I am, three weeks away from holding my book in my hands. It seems surreal. After I fell in February 2014, I could never have imagined this moment in time. *I believe everything happens for a reason, and I'm glad this is my reason.*

Resources

Here is a small list of resources. These are sites that I have
found helpful in my recovery, plus the one I created. I hope
that they steer you in the right direction.

Brain Injury Association of America
www.biausa.org

Brain Injury Alliance (each state has one, I am listing the Minnesota site)
www.braininjurymn.org

Brain Line
www.brainline.org

TBI Hope & Inspiration (sign up for their free digital magazine)
www.tbihopeandinspiration.com

Brain Injury Radio
www.blogtalkradio.com/braininjuryradio

Traumatic Brain Injury Survival Guide
www.tbiguide.com

Facebook ~ The TBI Tribe
https://www.facebook.com/groups/792052120888627/

Faces of TBI
www.facesoftbi.com

My doctors, clinics, and other resources in Minnesota:
Dr. Fred Clary, D.C., D.I.B.C.N.
Chiropractic Neurologist
www.afunctionallife.com

Dr. Robert Hardy, Ed.D.
Licensed Psychologist
www.afunctionallife.com

Greg Santema, PT
Cranial Sacral Therapy and Physical Therapy
www.novacare.com

James M. Mitchell, M.D.
Neuro Ophthalmologist
www.mccanneleye.com

National Dizzy & Balance Center
www.stopdizziness.com

Heuer Lund Flores, PA
Personal Injury Law
www.callhlf.com

Traumatic Brain Injury Center
http://www.hcmc.org/clinics/TraumaticBrainInjuryCenter/HCMC_CLINICS_448

Courage Kenny Rehabilitation
http://www.allinahealth.org/Courage-Kenny-Rehabilitation-Institute/

About the Author

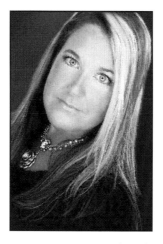

Photo by Krish Kiefer

Amy sustained her TBI in February of 2014 after falling on a patch of ice and landing full-force on the back of her skull. She is still recovering, and understanding the full scope of her injury. She is an author, professional photographer, and creative coach located in Saint Paul, MN. She is a frequent contributor to *The Huffington Post,* and a loud and proud advocate for TBI awareness. She travels the country with her Yorkie, Pixxie, and brings awareness everywhere she goes.

She is currently working on her second book, *Faces of TBI.* Amy is available for speaking at conferences and events, and may be reached by email: AmyZellmerTBI@gmail.com

She believes that the healing process begins with the telling of your story, releasing everything that you've been bottling up inside. Her goal is to tell other survivors' stories. TBI is an invisible disability that many don't understand. She wants to bring an awareness and understanding to the world, and hopes that people will have more compassion for those who look seemingly fine—but inside are struggling with memory or cognitive issues, such as she is.

Amy is addicted to Starbucks, Miss Me Jeans, chocolate, and all things pink and glittery.

Connect with Amy:
www.facesoftbi.com
www.facebook.com/facesoftbi
www.twitter.com/amyzellmer
www.instagram.com/amyzellmer